Pelvic Floor Exercises for Seniors

A Comprehensive Workout Guide to Heal Sexual Dysfunctions, Incontinences, Pains, Prolapses and Muscle Weakening

Peter Michtor

Table of Contents

Introduction

Our bodies are the loom in the fabric of life, weaving the complex threads of experiences, resiliency, and time. The golden years beckon with the promise of knowledge, deep connections, and a depth of insight that only time can impart as we journey through the chapters of our existence. However, the physical complexities of aging can occasionally throw shade on the vibrant picture, impacting our wellness from the very core. At this point, the pelvic floor, an often-overlooked element of health comes into sharp focus.

Welcome to "Pelvic Floor Exercises for Seniors: This book is a beacon of empowerment that will lead you on a transforming journey to strengthen and reclaim your pelvic floor, an essential component of your overall health. It is more than just a compilation of exercises.

The pelvic floor is a cornerstone in the mosaic of human anatomy, supporting the complex network of organs within the pelvis and essential to the preservation of balance, core strength, and grounded vitality. Like every other aspect of our body, the pelvic floor changes as we age gracefully. These changes can show up as weaker muscles, less control over one's bladder, or problems that affect one's mental and physical health, among other manifestations.

The author has thoughtfully and carefully considered the special requirements of elderly readers, addressing potential obstacles and offering a path forward to promote resilience, strength, and overall well-being. We start by delving into the pelvic floor and attempting to piece together its anatomy and function. You will gain an understanding of the importance of this sometimes-underappreciated bodily part through explanations given.

The activities in this guide are what really make it worthwhile. They have been carefully chosen and tailored to meet the various needs of seniors. Every exercise is provided with clarity and precision, to enable accessibility for anyone, regardless of experience level or recent start-up in wellness.

"Pelvic Floor Exercises for Seniors" explores the psychological and emotional aspects of pelvic health in addition to the physical. An integrated viewpoint that emphasizes the connection of the mind, body, and spirit is provided through expert insights, real-life testimonies, and interviews with medical specialists.

Join us as we take you on a life-changing journey via the pages of this book, which will serve as a guide to improved health, regenerated energy, and a closer relationship with your own body.

Learn to love being active, to be resilient, and to feel the tremendous effects of having a healthy pelvic floor on your overall well-being. May the chapters provide you with motivation, direction, and a fresh feeling of self-efficacy as you travel toward the golden years of maximum health and vitality.

Understanding the Importance of Pelvic Floor Exercises for Seniors

The human body undergoes several changes as we age, and one vital but frequently disregarded development is the state of the pelvic floor. Organs include the bladder, uterus (in women), and rectum receive vital support from the complex network of muscles, ligaments, and tissues that makes up the pelvic floor. Maintaining the pelvic floor's strength and functionality as seniors age into their golden years is increasingly important for general wellbeing. This comprehensive note seeks to clarify the importance of pelvic floor exercises for seniors and guide them through a thorough comprehension of the activities that can improve their quality of life and overall health.

1. Anatomy and Function of the Pelvic Floor:

At the base of the pelvis, a group of muscles comprise the pelvic floor, which resembles a hammock. It is essential for sustaining continence, supporting the organs, and adding stability to the core. Controlling bowel and bladder function, supporting the spine, and facilitating sexual function are all made possible by the pelvic floor muscles.

2. Age-Related Changes in the Pelvic Floor:

Hormonal fluctuations, childbirth (for women), and normal tissue aging can cause the pelvic floor muscles to decrease with age. Problems like pelvic organ prolapse, urine incontinence, and diminished sexual function could arise from this weakening. Exercises for the pelvic floor provide a proactive, non-invasive way to deal with and avoid these issues.

3. Benefits of Pelvic Floor Exercises for Seniors:

a. Better Bladder Control: Consistent pelvic floor exercises help strengthen and better coordinate the muscles in charge of bladder control, which lowers the risk of urine incontinence.

b. Improved Sexual performance: By boosting muscular tone and blood flow to the pelvic area, strengthening the pelvic floor can help with enhanced sexual performance.

c. Preventing Pelvic Organ Prolapse: Specific exercises lower the risk of pelvic organ prolapse by preserving the integrity of the pelvic floor support structures.

d. Posture and Core Stability: A strong pelvic floor is essential to core stability, which improves posture and overall stability, both of which are crucial in later life.

e. Reduction of Lower Back Pain: By supporting the lower back, strengthening the pelvic floor may help reduce pain and discomfort brought on by aging-related changes.

4. Pelvic Floor Exercises for Seniors:

a. Kegel exercises: These help to develop control and strength by alternating between contraction and relaxation of the pelvic floor muscles. Kegel exercises can be gradually increased in difficulty based on a person's current fitness level.

b. Bridge Exercises: Strengthening the glutes, hamstrings, and lower back while doing bridge exercises enhances overall stability by activating the core and pelvic floor.

c. Deep Abdominal Breathing: Using diaphragmatic breathing exercises will help you become more relaxed and flexible while also raising your awareness of your pelvic floor.

d. Pelvic tilts: By gently tilting the pelvis back and forth, these exercises activate the pelvic floor and increase lower back flexibility.

5. Seeking Professional Advice:

Although pelvic floor exercises have advantages, seniors should always seek the advice of healthcare providers, such as physical therapists or pelvic floor specialists, for specific advice. These experts are capable of evaluating each person's needs, creating customized workout plans, and taking care of any underlying medical issues.

Pelvic floor exercises for Seniors are essential to proactive, all-encompassing health care. These activities can help seniors maintain their independence, build strength, and improve their general quality of life when incorporated into a regular program. It is never too late to make an investment in pelvic floor health, and seniors can take a journey towards ongoing wellbeing and vitality with the correct information and dedication.

Essential Needs for Pelvic Floor Exercises for Seniors

The path of aging is one of great wonder, characterized by the accumulation of life's subtleties, wisdom, and experiences. But even as the years gracefully pass, the complex network of physical changes can throw a shadow over the good times, posing particular difficulties that need for careful consideration. The pelvic floor is one of the most important but frequently disregarded parts of senior health that needs to be understood and taken care of. We examine the particular requirements that make pelvic floor exercises essential for seniors in this in-depth note.

1. Weakening and Atrophy of Muscles:

Physical Changes: Natural physiological changes brought on by aging cause a progressive decrease of muscular mass and strength, including the pelvic floor muscles.

Effect on the Pelvic Floor: With time, the pelvic floor muscles which support the bladder, uterus, and rectum may weaken and become less effective. This could result in problems like incontinence, prolapse of the pelvic organs, and decreased sexual function.

2. Sustaining Bladder Control:

Prevalence of Incontinence: Urinary incontinence is a prevalent problem among the seniors. Pelvic floor exercises are essential for improving bladder control because they strengthen the muscles involved in continence.

Exercise-Based Empowerment: Seniors can restore control over their bladder function by performing targeted pelvic floor exercises, which lessens the negative effects of incontinence on everyday activities and overall quality of life.

3. Supporting Sexual Health:

The Pelvic Floor's Function in Intimacy: The pelvic floor is essential for arousal, sensation, and orgasm in sexual activity. Sexual health may vary as people age, and pelvic floor exercises can help preserve or restore intimate well-being.

Increasing Sensation: Exercises that improve pelvic blood flow, muscle tone, and flexibility can boost one's sexual satisfaction and self-esteem and encourage a positive outlook on intimacy as one ages.

4. Preventing Pelvic Organ Prolapse:

Identifying Prolapse: Pelvic organ prolapse is a disorder in which the organs of the pelvis descend as a result of compromised support structures. Seniors may be more vulnerable, especially ladies who have just given birth.

Strengthening Support Structures: By strengthening the muscles and connective tissues that support the pelvic organs, pelvic floor exercises serve as a preventive measure and lower the chance of prolapse and the discomfort that comes with it.

5. Handling Chronic Pain and Discomfort:

Difficulties with Chronic Pain: Elderly people may have persistent pelvic pain or discomfort, which is frequently associated with diseases like arthritis, inflammation, or previous accidents.

Relieving Pain: By increasing blood flow, strengthening muscular support, and increasing range of motion, targeted workouts can reduce pain and promote comfort and wellness.

6. Improving Posture and Stability:

Essential Function of the Pelvic Floor: A crucial component of the core muscles, the pelvic floor aids with posture and general stability.

Reducing Fall Risk: Exercises that strengthen the pelvic floor help seniors keep their balance, lower their chance of falling, and improve their general mobility.

The requirements for pelvic floor workouts become apparent as an essential threads in the complex tapestry of senior health, interlacing vitality, wellness, and self-assurance. Seniors who accept the empowering path of focused exercises take a step toward addressing the unique needs of the pelvic floor and toward a more vibrant, holistic approach to aging gracefully.

Factors to Consider

Setting out on a path toward senior pelvic floor health involves a comprehension of a number of variables. Exercise concerns become more crucial as the body ages gracefully in order to guarantee both safety and efficacy. This extensive manual explores the various issues that seniors should take into account when performing pelvic floor exercises. A customized and comprehensive approach to pelvic floor health is shaped by a variety of factors, from medical and physical concerns to emotional and psychological components.

1. Physical Health Assessment:

Seniors should have a comprehensive physical health evaluation performed by a licensed healthcare provider prior to beginning any pelvic floor exercise program. Evaluations of joint flexibility, muscle strength, and general physical health may be part of this assessment.

Exercise programs must take into account previous illnesses, such as osteoporosis, arthritis, or musculoskeletal problems, in order to be customized for each user.

2. Medication and Medical History:

It's critical to comprehend the senior's medication history. Exercise decisions may be impacted by health conditions including diabetes, hypertension, or cardiovascular problems.

Certain drugs have the potential to affect fluid balance or muscle tone, which could impact how well pelvic floor exercises work. It is necessary to speak with a healthcare professional in order to modify exercises appropriately.

3. Mobility and Range of Motion:

The mobility and range of motion of seniors may change. Exercise modifications should take into account the person's mobility aids and any restrictions on joint flexibility.

Stretching plans and other mild activities that increase flexibility can improve pelvic floor health overall without putting too much strain on the body.

4. Cognitive Considerations:

The performance of exercises is influenced by cognitive health. Seniors can benefit from visual aids and clear, succinct directions to help them understand and correctly do pelvic floor exercises.

Exercises that are customized to a person's cognitive capacities guarantee participation and regimen adherence.

5. Emotional and Psychological Wellbeing:

Stress and anxiety are two examples of emotional variables that might affect pelvic floor health. Physical activities can be enhanced by mindbody practices like mindfulness and relaxation techniques.

Fostering a healthy mental attitude requires open communication with healthcare practitioners, resolving concerns, and setting reasonable expectations.

6. Social Support:

When there is social support, pelvic floor exercises can be more pleasurable and long-lasting. Seniors who are encouraged to join in classes or group activities feel more motivated and part of the community.

Environments that are supportive can help people maintain their workout plan and have a good outlook.

7. Progression and Gradual Intensity:

Seniors should be given time to get used to new motions and routines by introducing pelvic floor exercises gradually.

It's critical to track development and gradually increase or decrease intensity. Regular evaluations by medical experts guarantee that physical activities continue to be safe and helpful.

8. Nutrition and Hydration:

Sufficient nutrition and hydration are essential for maintaining general health, which includes the health of muscles and connective tissues.

Pelvic floor exercises are more effective when done in conjunction with a well-balanced diet high in nutrients, particularly those that support bone and muscle health.

9. Regular Monitoring and Feedback:

Based on progress or modifications in health status, regular check-ins with healthcare practitioners enable modifications to the exercise program.

Giving input on how comfortable you feel and whether you experience any pain or discomfort while exercising helps customize the routine to meet your needs.

A comprehensive strategy that takes into account the complex interactions between physical, physiological, mental, and social issues is crucial when designing a pelvic floor exercise program for seniors.

Seniors can start a road toward pelvic floor health that is not only effective but also long-lasting and rewarding, improving their general well-being and quality of life, by acknowledging and taking care of these factors.

Nutrients Required

It's important for seniors starting pelvic floor exercises to understand that sustaining total health and wellbeing involves more than just physical activity. To maximize the advantages of pelvic floor exercises and maintain the body's resilience, a comprehensive strategy incorporating appropriate nutrition is needed. The nutrients listed below are essential for supporting seniors' pelvic floor health:

1. Protein:

A vital nutrition for seniors performing pelvic floor exercises, protein is necessary for both muscle maintenance and healing.

Consume foods high in lean protein, such as fish, poultry, lentils, and dairy products, to aid in the growth and repair of muscles, particularly the pelvic floor muscles.

2. Calcium:

Bone health is mostly dependent on calcium, and strong bones are necessary for pelvic floor stability.

Include dairy products, leafy greens, and plant-based milk that has been fortified in your diet to make sure you are getting enough calcium.

3. Magnesium:

Although it's sometimes disregarded, magnesium is vital for relaxed muscles, which is necessary for pelvic floor exercises.

Consume whole grains, nuts, seeds, and leafy green vegetables to keep your magnesium levels at their ideal range.

4. Vitamin D:

In order to maintain bone health and muscle function, vitamin D and calcium work in concert.

Good sources of vitamin D include dairy products fortified with vitamin D, sunshine exposure, and fatty seafood like salmon.

5. Fiber:

Eating a diet high in fiber encourages regular bowel movements, and constipation can aggravate pelvic floor problems.

To keep your digestive system healthy, include entire grains, fruits, vegetables, and legumes.

6. Hydration:

Maintaining enough hydration is essential for general health and can help avoid the problems with urine that come with pelvic floor dysfunction.

Drink plenty of water throughout the day, and include items high in water content in your meals, such as fruits and vegetables.

7. Omega 3 Fatty Acids:

These vital fatty acids promote cardiovascular health, which is linked to pelvic floor function, and have anti-inflammatory qualities.

For a good supply of omega-3 fatty acids, incorporate walnuts, chia seeds, flaxseeds, and fatty fish into your diet.

8. Vitamin C:

Vitamin C supports collagen, which is necessary to keep connective tissues intact.

Vitamin C is abundant in citrus fruits, berries, and vegetables like bell peppers.

9. Zinc:

Zinc is necessary for immune system and tissue healing as well as general health, which includes pelvic floor wellness.

Include foods high in zinc in your diet, such as dairy, meat, nuts, and seeds.

10. Probiotics:

Digestion is aided by probiotics, and a healthy gut is associated with overall wellness.

Incorporate probiotic-rich foods such as kefir, sauerkraut, and yogurt to support a healthy gut microbiome.

Pelvic Floor Exercises for Incontinences

1. Pelvic Tilt:

Instructions:

Position yourself comfortably in a sitting or lying position with your knees bent and your feet flat on the ground.

Breathe in and push your lower back against the surface while bending your pelvis slightly backward.

Exhale and return to the neutral position.

Repeat 10-15 times, gradually increasing the number each time you get more comfortable.

2. Kegel Exercises:

Instructions:

Comfortably lie down or sit.

Squeeze your vaginal and anus muscles as though you're attempting to halt the flow of urine.

After five seconds of holding, release, and relax.

Repeat 10-15 times, progressively extending the hold period.

3. Bridge Exercise:

Instructions:

Position yourself on your back with your knees bent and your feet flat on the ground.

Using your pelvic floor and glutes, take a deep breath and raise your hips toward the ceiling.

Hold for a short while before letting go and bringing your hips down.

Do this 10-12 times.

4. Seated Marching:

Instructions:

With your feet flat on the ground, take a seat in a sturdy chair.

Raise one knee to your chest and keep it there for a short while.

Repeat with the other knee after lowering the leg.

10-15 repetitions of alternating legs should be performed.

5. Butterfly Stretch:

Instructions:

Position yourself on the floor with your feet flat on the ground.

Gently press your knees toward the floor while using your hands to hold your feet.

Hold while taking deep breaths for 15-30 seconds.

6. Ball Squeeze:

Instructions:

Take a comfortable seat on a stability ball or chair.

A small, soft ball should be placed between your knees.

Using your knees, squeeze the ball and hold it for five seconds.

After releasing, carry out 10-15 repetitions.

7. Standing Pelvic Clocks:

Instructions:

Feet should be hip-width apart.

Tilt your pelvis forward to the twelve, three, six, and nine o'clock positions, as if there were a floor clock.

After 12 minutes of steadily moving in a circle, reverse your direction.

8. Pelvic Floor Relaxation Stretch:

Instructions:

As you sit comfortably, inhale deeply a few times.

Consciously relax your pelvic floor muscles as you release the breath.

After 10 seconds of holding the relaxed position, repeat for 10 breath cycles.

9. Supine Hip Abduction:

Instructions:

Position yourself on your back with your feet flat on the floor and your knees bent.

While keeping your feet together, extend your knees outward.

After a brief period of holding, go back to the initial position.

Do this 10-12 times.

10. Pelvic Floor Drops:

Instructions:

Take a seat comfortably in a chair or stability ball.

Breathe in, and then release it while contracting your pelvic floor muscles slightly.

Let go and completely relax the muscles.

Concentrate on controlled contraction and release as you repeat for 10-15 cycles.

Pelvic Floor Exercises for Prolapses

1. Pelvic Floor Contractions:

Instructions:

Comfortably lie down or sit.

Breathe deeply in, and then gently contract your pelvic floor muscles as you release the breath.

For five counts, hold the contraction.

Relax and repeat 10-15 times, progressively lengthening the hold.

2. Wall Sit with Pelvic Floor Engagement:

Instructions:

Place your feet shoulder-width apart and lean your back against a wall.

To get into a sitting position, slide down the wall.

Hold the wall sit position for 20-30 seconds while contracting your pelvic floor muscles.

Get to your feet slowly and repeat 10-12 times.

3. Pelvic Tilt on Stability Ball:

Instructions:

With your feet flat on the ground, take a seat on a stability ball.

Take a breath, tuck your pelvis back, and push your lower back against the ball.

Take a breath out and come back to neutral.

Concentrate on controlled movements as you repeat 10-15 times.

4. Modified Bridge Workout:

Instructions:

With your feet flat on the ground and your knees bent, lie on your back.

Taking a deep breath, raise your hips and contract your pelvic floor and glutes.

Hold for a short while before letting go and bringing your hips down.

Concentrating on keeping the pelvic floor engaged, repeat 10-12 times.

5. Deep Squats with Pelvic Floor Focus:

Instructions:

Place your feet shoulder-width apart as you stand.

Keeping your back straight and your chest raised, lower yourself into a deep squat.

As you return to standing, contract your pelvic floor muscles.

Concentrating on the connection between your pelvic floor and squat movement, repeat 10-12 times.

6. Side-lying Leg Lifts:

Instructions:

With your legs straight, lie on your side.

Raise the upper leg while maintaining an engaged pelvic floor.

After 10-12 repetitions on each side, lower the leg.

7. Pelvic Clocks in Side-lying Position:

Instructions:

Bend your knees slightly while lying on your side.

Picture a clock on the ground below you.

Lift your top knee, creating a circular motion like the hands of a clock.

Spend 12 minutes in each direction rotating in a circular manner, focus on pelvic floor engagement and strengthening.

8. Seated Leg Press with Pelvic Floor Emphasis:

Instructions:

Place your back against a supportive chair to provide comfort.

Engage the pelvic floor by straightening one leg in front of you.

After a short while of holding, lower the leg.

On each leg, perform 10-12 repetitions.

9. Pelvic Floor Stretch with Deep Breathing:

Instructions:

With your feet flat on the ground, take a seat on a chair's edge.

Take a deep breath and lengthen your spine.

Breathe out while extending your pelvic floor with a slight forward bend.

Hold for 15-30 seconds while concentrating on relaxation.

10. Modified Child's Pose:

Instructions:

Place yourself on your hands and knees like you're on a table.

With your arms out in front of you, take a seat back onto your heels.

Lean your chest gently to the floor so that your pelvic floor can expand.

Hold for 15-30 seconds while taking deep breaths and letting go of the tension.

Note: Although the specific needs of people with prolapses are taken into account when designing these exercises, special considerations and changes may be required depending on the severity of the problem.

Always pay attention to your body's signals and move at a safe and comfortable speed.

Pelvic Floor Exercises against Falls

1. Heel Raises with Pelvic Floor Engagement:

Instructions:

Feets should be hip-width apart.

Lift yourself onto the balls of your feet by gradually raising your heels off the ground.

As you raise and lower your heels, contract your pelvic floor muscles.

With an emphasis on preserving balance and pelvic floor engagement, repeat 10-15 times.

2. Single-Leg Balance:

Instructions:

If you need assistance, stand close to a stable surface.

Raise one leg and balance on it while bending at the knee.

For 10-15 seconds, contract and hold your pelvic floor muscles.

Continue with the opposite leg, progressively lengthening the reps as your strength improves.

3. Tai Chi Inspired Weight Shifts:

Instructions:

Stand with feet shoulder-width apart.

Gently transfer your weight from one leg to the other while using deliberate, gradual motions.

Maintain a contracted pelvic floor as you shift weight.

Concentrate on balance and stability during the 12-minute performance.

4. Sit-to-Stand Exercises:

Instructions:

Feet flat on the ground, take a seat in a firm chair.

Employing your pelvic floor and leg muscles, carefully stand up.

Return to your seat with control.

Repeat 10-12 times, emphasizing proper form and balance.

5. Marching in Place:

Instructions:

Feet should be hip-width apart.

While you march in place, lift your knees.

With every lift, contract your pelvic floor.

Maintain your concentrate on balance and deliberate movements for the next 12 minutes.

6. Toe Taps:

Instructions:

Place your feet hip-width apart.

Lift one foot and tap your toe to the side, then bring it back to center.

Put your pelvic floor into action and switch sides.

Do this 10-15 times on each side.

7. Sideways Walking:

Instructions:

Make use of a room that is clear and open.

As you move sideways, contract your pelvic floor muscles.

Keep going for 12 minutes, paying attention to your stability and balance.

8. Calf Raises with Pelvic Floor Activation:

Instructions:

Feet should be hip-width apart.

Lift onto your toes, engaging your pelvic floor as you rise.

Return to lowering your heels.

Focusing on balance and pelvic floor engagement, repeat 10-15 times.

9. Modified Yoga Tree Pose:

Instructions:

Step up close to a sturdy object.

Place the sole of your other foot on your inner thigh or calf and shift your weight to that leg.

For 15-30 seconds, contract and hold your pelvic floor.

On the other leg, repeat.

10. Back Leg Raises:

Instructions:

Grasp a sturdy chair for support while you stand behind it.

Lift one leg back straight back while engaging your pelvic floor.

Repeat on the other side after lowering the leg.

On each leg, perform 10-15 lifts, paying attention to your balance and muscular activation.

Before beginning any exercise program, especially for seniors who are worried about falling, speak with a trained fitness instructor or healthcare provider. Although the purpose of these exercises is to increase stability and balance, depending on one's fitness level and overall health, adjustments and considerations may need to be made.

Pelvic Floor Exercises against Muscle Weakening

1. Seated Pelvic Tilts:

Instructions:

With your back straight, take a comfortable seat.

Take a breath and arch your lower back by tilting your pelvis forward.

As you round your lower back and tilt your pelvis backward, release the breath.

For 10-15 repetitions, repeat this movement, paying attention to the controlled, gentle tilting.

2. The Butterfly Stretch:

Instructions:

With your feet flat on the ground, take a seat.

Gently press your knees toward the floor while using your hands to hold your feet.

Breathe deeply while holding the stretch for 15-30 seconds.

For increased pelvic floor engagement and flexibility, release and repeat.

3. Pelvic Floor Contractions:

Instructions:

Comfortably lie down or sit.

Breathe deeply in, and then tense your pelvic floor muscles as you release the breath.

After holding the contraction for 5 counts, release it.

Repeat 10-15 times, progressively extending the hold period.

4. Modified Bridge Exercise:

Instructions:

With your feet flat on the ground and your knees bent, lie on your back.

Using your pelvic floor and glutes, take a deep breath and raise your hips toward the ceiling.

Hold for a short while before letting go and bringing your hips down.

To strengthen the surrounding muscles and pelvic floor, repeat 10-12 times.

5. Seated Pelvic Clocks:

Instructions:

Take a comfortable chair.

Tilt your pelvis forward, to the sides, backward, and to the opposite side in a circular motion, as if there were a clock beneath you.

For 12 minutes, focus on making slow, deliberate rotations while performing this exercise.

6. Leg Slides:

Instructions:

Place your feet flat on the floor and bend your knees while lying on your back.

Straighten your leg and slowly glide one foot along the floor.

Restore your leg to its initial position by using your pelvic floor.

For 10-15 repetitions, switch to the other leg and repeat with it.

7. Seated Marching:

Instructions:

With your feet flat on the ground, take a seat in a sturdy chair.

Raise one knee to your chest and keep it there for a short while.

Repeat with the other knee after lowering the leg.

10-15 repetitions of alternating legs should be performed.

8. Supine Knee Drops:

Instructions:

With your feet flat on the ground and your knees bent, lie on your back.

Drop one knee slowly to the side to activate the pelvic floor.

Return the knee to the middle, and then switch to the opposite side.

Repeat 10-15 times on each side.

9. Inner Thigh Squeeze:

Instructions:

Maintain a straight back as you sit in a chair.

Stuff a cushion or soft ball between your inner thighs.

Squeeze the ball while using your pelvic floor and inner thighs.

Repeat 10-15 times by holding for 5 seconds, letting go, and repeating.

10. Pelvic Floor Relaxation Stretch:

Instructions:

As you sit comfortably, inhale deeply a few times.

Consciously relax your pelvic floor muscles as you release the breath.

After ten seconds of holding the relaxed position, repeat for ten breath cycles.

Multipurpose Pelvic Floor Exercises for Seniors

It is also applied in sexual health issues

1. Kegel Exercises:

Instructions:

Comfortably lie down or sit.

Squeeze your vaginal and anus muscles as though you're attempting to halt the flow of pee.

After five seconds of holding, release, and relax.

Repeat 10-15 times, progressively extending the hold period.

2. Pelvic Tilt with Breathwork:

Instructions:

With your feet flat on the ground and your knees bent, lie on your back.

Take a deep breath and lift your pelvis.

Let go of the breath and let your lower back gently contact the ground.

Repeat 10-12 times, paying attention to pelvic movement and relaxation.

3. The Butterfly Stretch:

Instructions:

With your feet flat on the ground, sit on the floor.

Gently press your knees toward the floor while using your hands to hold your feet.

Breathe deeply while holding the stretch for 15-30 seconds.

In order to improve pelvic flexibility, release and repeat.

4. Seated Leg Lifts:

Instructions:

With your back erect, take a seat in a firm chair.

Straighten one leg in front of you while using your pelvic floor.

After a short while, release the leg.

Repeat 10-15 lifts with the other leg.

5. The Hip Flexor Stretch:

Instructions:

With your other foot in front, make a 90-degree angle and kneel on one knee.

Push your hips forward gently until you feel a stretch in the pelvic area.

After holding for 15-30 seconds, switch legs.

6. CatCow Stretch:

Instructions:

Place yourself on your hands and knees like you're a table.

Breathe in while arching your back (cow pose).

Exhale while tucking your pelvis and rounding your back (cat pose).

To increase pelvic area flexibility, repeat for 10-12 cycles.

7. Bridge Pose:

Instructions:

Lie on your back with your knees bent and your feet flat on the ground.

Engage your pelvic floor as you take a breath and raise your hips toward the ceiling.

Hold for a short while before letting go and bringing your hips down.

To strengthen the pelvic muscles, repeat 10-12 times.

8. Deep Squats:

Instructions:

Position yourself so that your feet are shoulder-width apart.

Squat down deeply while using your pelvic floor.

Rise back to the standing position.

Continue doing 10-12 squats, paying attention to pelvic engagement.

9. Pelvic Clocks in Supine Position:

Instructions:

Bend your knees and lie on your back.

Make a circular movement with your pelvis while visualizing a clock underneath you.

Do this for 12 minutes to improve your pelvic mobility.

10. Inner Thigh Squeeze with Breathwork:

Instructions:

Maintain a straight back as you sit in a chair.

Stuff a cushion or soft ball between your inner thighs.

Squeeze the ball, inhale, and hold it for five seconds.

Breathe out and then back in, repeating 10-15 times.

11. Pelvic Floor Relaxation with Meditation:

Instructions:

Close your eyes and take a comfortable seat.

Breathe deeply and see your pelvic area becoming less tense.

Let go of any residual stress by exhaling.

Repeat mixing mindfulness and relaxation for ten minutes.

12. Seated Pelvic Circles:

Instructions:

Take a comfortable chair.

Start with a gentle one-way circle and work your way around to the other.

To encourage pelvic flexibility, perform for 23 minutes.

13. Side-Lying Leg Lifts:

Instructions:

With your legs straight, lie on your side.

Raise your upper leg while using your pelvic floor.

After 10-15 repetitions on each side, lower the leg.

14. Child's Pose with Breathwork:

Instructions:

Begin on the hands and knees position and then return to your heels.

Take a deep breath and feel your pelvis expand.

Let out the breath and let your chest descend to the floor.

Repeat for 10-12 breath cycles.

15. Seated Twist:

Instructions:

Position yourself so that your legs are out in front of you.

Hugging the knee, cross one leg over the other.

Lengthening your spine with an inhaled breath, release it with a slight twist.

To improve the flexibility and mobility of the pelvis, hold for 15-30 seconds on each side.

16. Pelvic Floor Activated Leg Press:

Instructions:

Sit or lie down with knees bent.

Engaging your pelvic floor, press one foot into the ground.

After 5 seconds, release.

Perform 10-15 repetitions switching legs.

17. Ankle Circles with Pelvic Engagement:

Instructions:

Take a seat with your feet lifted off the ground.

Rotate one ankle around in a circle.

While you circle, engage your pelvic floor.

Change directions and repeat with the opposite ankle.

18. Lateral Leg Lifts with Standing:

Instructions:

For support, stand close to a solid surface.

Exert one leg to the side to activate the pelvic floor.

Lower, and then proceed to the opposite side.

Lift your legs 10-15 times each.

19. Pelvic Floor Contraction March:

Instructions:

Keep your back straight while you sit or stand.

March in place, focusing each step on contractions of the pelvic floor.

Keep going for 12 minutes, paying attention to your muscle engagement.

20. Pelvic Floor Relaxation with Deep Breaths:

Instructions:

Lie down comfortably.

Take a deep breath, expanding your diaphragm.

Release the tension in your pelvic floor by exhaling.

Repeat for 10 minutes, alternating between pelvic relaxation and deep breathing.

21. Diaphragmatic Breathing with Pelvic Floor Engagement:

Instructions:

With one hand on your chest and the other on your abdomen, take a comfortable seat.

Take a deep breath and let your diaphragm expand.

When you exhale, pull your navel into your spine and activate your pelvic floor.

Repeat 10-15 times using your breaths.

22. Standing Pelvic Clocks:

Instructions:

Feet should be hip-width apart.

Imagine a floor-based clock, and make circular movements with your pelvis.

For 23 minutes, make both clockwise and counterclockwise circles.

23. Pelvic Floor Lifts on Stability Ball:

Instructions:

With your feet flat on the ground, take a seat on a stability ball.

Engage your pelvic floor by raising your hips toward the ceiling.

After a short while, release and lower.

Repeat for 10-12 lifts.

24. Heel Slides:

Instructions:

Bend your knees and lie on your back.

To straighten the leg, slide one heel along the floor.

Put your pelvic floor into action and take a step back to the starting position.

Repeat on each leg for 10-15 slides.

25. Standing Leg Abduction:

Instructions:

Stand near a sturdy surface.

Exert one leg to the side to engage the pelvic floor.

Lower after 5 seconds of holding.

10-15 repetitions on the other leg.

26. Seated Pelvic Floor Twists:

Instructions:

Maintain a straight back as you sit in a chair.

Turn your body to one side so that your pelvic floor is activated.

After holding for 10-15 seconds, rotate to the opposite side.

27. Pelvic Body Drops on Stability Ball:

Instructions:

With your feet flat on the ground, take a seat on a stability ball.

Breathe in, contract your pelvic floor, and then let go of the breath.

Repeat 10-15 times, paying attention to your controlled motions.

28. Clamshell Exercise:

Instructions:

Bend your knees and lie on your side.

Raise your upper leg while using your pelvic floor.

Repeat lowering the knee after 10-15 lifts on each side.

29. Standing Pelvic Flexibility Stretch:

Instructions:

Feet should be hip-width apart.

Reaching toward the floor, bend forward at the hips.

Let your pelvis relax and hold it there for 15-30 seconds.

30. Pelvic Floor Activation during Daily Activities:

Instructions:

While performing daily duties, work on using your pelvic floor.

For increased strength and awareness, deliberately contract and release these muscles when standing, sitting, or walking throughout the day.

These exercises include a variety of motions to treat seniors' pelvic floor health. Before starting any workout regimen, always get medical advice, especially if you have any particular health issues.

Its Effectiveness

Pelvic floor exercises play a crucial role in preventing falls and injuries among seniors by contributing to overall stability, balance, and core strength. Here are key aspects of their effectiveness:

1. Better Balance: Using the core muscles, which include those that support the pelvis, is a common aspect of pelvic floor exercises. A stronger core results in improved balance, which lowers the chance of falling.

2. Enhanced Stability: Improving pelvic floor strength enhances stability in general. Seniors who have a firm base are less likely to experience abrupt falls by maintaining their equilibrium during a variety of activities.

3. Enhanced Muscle Tone: By focusing on and fortifying particular muscle groups, pelvic floor exercises enhance the tone of the muscles in the pelvic area. Better organ support from this increased tone promotes stability and reduces the risk of harm.

4. Prevention of Pelvic Organ Prolapse: It is well recognized that pelvic floor exercises can assist in managing and preventing pelvic organ prolapse. Seniors can lessen their chance of organ descent, which can cause pain and imbalance, by strengthening their pelvic muscles and connective tissues.

5. Improved Gait and Mobility: Good posture and body alignment are supported by a healthy pelvic floor, which has a beneficial effect on gait and general mobility. Increased mobility in seniors lowers their risk of falling because they are less likely to trip or stumble.

6. Bladder and Bowel Control: Pelvic floor exercises help lessen the need to hurriedly visit the restroom by enhancing bladder and bowel control. Increased control over these processes leads to more purposeful movements and reduces the chance of falls brought on by unexpected bursts of energy.

7. Beneficial Effect on Bone Health: Weightlifting activities, which are frequently a part of pelvic floor regimens, are beneficial for bone density. Stronger bones help the body sustain itself more effectively and lower the chance of fractures in the event of a fall.

8. Fall Prevention Programs: Comprehensive fall prevention programs for seniors usually include pelvic floor exercises. To address different components of fall risk, these programs usually combine strength training, balancing exercises, and flexibility routines.

9. Enhanced Confidence: Seniors who engage in pelvic floor exercises report feeling more confident in their ability to move and carry out everyday tasks as a result of their improved strength and control. Increased self-assurance can result in more solid and safe movements, which lowers the chance of falls.

10. Mind-Body link: Pelvic floor exercises help promote awareness of posture and body movements by incorporating a mind-body link. This increased awareness can help prevent falls by being proactive in averting potentially dangerous circumstances.

In conclusion, including pelvic floor exercises to an all-encompassing senior fitness program can help significantly reduce the risk of falls and injuries.

When combined with a comprehensive fitness program, these exercises help seniors live better by improving their strength, stability, and general health, which lowers their risk of injury and improves their quality of life.

Conclusion

The importance of pelvic floor exercises for seniors in the larger context of aging well and preserving optimal health cannot be emphasized. These workouts, which are sometimes disregarded in conventional fitness plans, turn out to be essential in addressing a wide range of physical issues related to aging, providing a thorough strategy that goes beyond the boundaries of particular health issues. Seniors who include pelvic floor exercises in their daily plan can reap numerous benefits that enhance not only their physical health but also their mental and social well-being.

Exercises for the pelvic floor, such as the mildly effective Kegels or the more dynamic pelvic tilts and bridges, are preventative measures against a variety of problems that the aging population faces. They are essential to fall prevention programs because they enhance muscle tone, stability, and balance. These exercises reduce the chance of falls and accidents by strengthening the core, giving seniors more self-assurance and independence as they go about their daily lives.

The beneficial effects on pelvic health include problems like prolapse of the pelvic organs and incontinence, giving seniors useful skills to prevent and manage these difficulties. The exercises provide people back control over their bodies, fostering a transformational feeling of dignity and quality of life.

Additionally, the comprehensive approach of pelvic floor exercises recognizes the connection between sexual, mental, and physical health. Seniors who participate in focused exercise develop a body-awareness that goes beyond the physical, creating a mind-body connection. This enhanced awareness leads to better posture, gait, and general mobility, which promotes the advantages of consistent exercise through a positive feedback loop.

Pelvic floor exercises provide sexual health, which is frequently a delicate and overlooked topic in conversations about senior well-being, the attention it deserves. These exercises help seniors have a happy and meaningful personal life by addressing concerns with arousal, sensation, and pelvic muscular strength. They also promote emotional connection and general well-being.

Promoting the use of pelvic floor exercises by seniors promotes a change in the way that people view aging in general society. It promotes a proactive, stereotype-busting, and socially-challenging attitude to fitness and wellness. Seniors who embrace pelvic floor exercises set off on a path of empowerment, proving that health, vitality, and strength are achievable at any age.

Redefining the narrative of aging requires us to acknowledge the importance of pelvic floor exercises for seniors as we manage the complications of an aging population. It is evidence of the human body's tenacity, the effectiveness of prophylactic treatment, and the life-changing potential of holistic medical methods. By raising awareness, educating the public, and incorporating these activities into seniors' daily plans, we can all work toward a paradigm change that views aging as a chance for development, vitality, and a satisfying quality of life.

BONUS

Body Building Diets

Healthy lipids for hormone production, a balance of carbohydrates for long-term energy, and sufficient protein for muscle repair are the main components of a bodybuilding diet designed to complement pelvic floor workouts. It's also critical to include meals high in vitamins and minerals, which promote bone health and general wellbeing. Here are ten diet recommendations, complete with recipes and Instructions:

1. Grilled Chicken Breast Salad:

Ingredients:

Olive oil, balsamic vinegar, cucumber, cherry tomatoes, lettuce, salt, chicken breast and pepper.

Instructions:

Cook the chicken breast completely on the grill.

In a bowl, mix the cucumber, cherry tomatoes, and chopped lettuce.

After slicing, arrange the grilled chicken over the salad.

Dress with salt, pepper, olive oil, and balsamic vinegar.

2. Quinoa and Vegetable Stir-fry:

Ingredients:

Quinoa, mixed veggies (carrots, broccoli, and bell peppers), tofu or chicken, sesame oil, ginger, garlic, and soy sauce.

Instructions:

Follow the directions on the package to cook the quinoa.

Add sesame oil, ginger, garlic, and mixed vegetables to a stir-fried pan with chicken or tofu.

Mix in the soy sauce and cooked quinoa thoroughly.

3. Salmon and Sweet Potato:

Ingredients:

Lemon, olive oil, salt, pepper, asparagus, sweet potato and salmon fillet.

Instructions:

Squeeze lemon juice, salt, and pepper on the salmon and bake or grill it.

Toss asparagus and sweet potatoes in olive oil and roast.

Arrange the roasted sweet potatoes and asparagus as a bed for the salmon.

4. Egg and Spinach Omelette:

Ingredients:

Eggs, spinach, tomatoes, feta cheese, olive oil, salt, and pepper.

Instructions:

Eggs should be whisked and then added to a hot pan with olive oil.

Add the diced tomatoes, crumbled feta cheese, and spinach.

Fold the omelette, after folding, cook the omelette until the eggs are set through.

5. Greek Yogurt Parfait:

Ingredients:

Honey, granola, mixed berries (strawberries, blueberries), and Greek yogurt.

Instructions:

Arrange granola, mixed berries, and Greek yogurt in a glass.

Pour some honey over the top for further sweetness.

6. Turkey and Avocado Wrap:

Ingredients:

Avocado, lettuce, tomato, Greek yogurt, mustard, and turkey slices and wholegrain wrap.

Instructions:

Place the wholegrain wrapper out.

Spread mustard and Greek yogurt.

Arrange tomato, lettuce, avocado, and turkey slices in layers.

Tightly wrap and enjoy.

7. Cottage Cheese and Fruit Bowl:

Ingredients:

Almonds, kiwi pieces, pineapple chunks, and cottage cheese.

Instructions:

Mix pineapple chunks and kiwi slices with cottage cheese.

Add some almonds on top for added crunch.

8. Beef and Vegetables Stir Fry:

Ingredients:

Broccoli, bell peppers, snap peas, ginger, garlic, and soy sauce in addition to lean beef strips.

Instructions:

Stir-fry ginger and garlic-studded beef strips until they turn brown.

Add the snap peas, bell peppers, and broccoli.

Add the soy sauce and stir until the vegetables are tender.

9. Quinoa with Oven-Baked Chicken:

Ingredients:

Lemon, olive oil, thyme, salt, pepper, chicken thighs, quinoa, cherry tomatoes, and zucchini.

Instructions:

Bake the chicken thighs with lemon, thyme, salt, and pepper in a preheated oven.

Roast the quinoa, zucchini, and cherry tomatoes with olive oil.

Arrange the chicken over a bed of veggies and roasted quinoa.

10. Tuna Salad Bowl:

Ingredients:

Mixed greens, chickpeas, cherry tomatoes, cucumber, feta cheese, olives, lemon, olive oil, salt, and pepper.

Instructions:

In a bowl, mix together tuna, cucumber, olives, feta cheese, cherry tomatoes, mixed greens, and chickpeas.

Add lemon, olive oil, salt, and pepper for dressing.

The nutritional balance offered by these diet recommendations supports both pelvic floor exercises and bodybuilding. Never forget to modify portion sizes according to your own nutritional requirements and fitness objectives.

Water consumption throughout the day is also crucial for maintaining general health and improving workout performance.

www.ingramcontent.com/pod-product-compliance
Lightning Source LLC
Chambersburg PA
CBHW061013260726
48661CB00005B/2180